YOUR KNOWLEDGE HAS VALUE

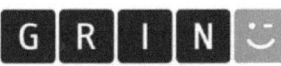

Bibliographic information published by the German National Library:

The German National Library lists this publication in the National Bibliography; detailed bibliographic data are available on the Internet at http://dnb.dnb.de .

Imprint:

Copyright © 2017 GRIN Verlag, Open Publishing GmbH
Print and binding: Books on Demand GmbH, Norderstedt Germany
ISBN: 9783668593244

This book at GRIN:

https://www.grin.com/document/383938

Diriba Legesse, Minda Garesu

Salmonella Enteritidis. Transovarial Transmission Meachanism in laying Chickens

GRIN Publishing

GRIN - Your knowledge has value

Since its foundation in 1998, GRIN has specialized in publishing academic texts by students, college teachers and other academics as e-book and printed book. The website www.grin.com is an ideal platform for presenting term papers, final papers, scientific essays, dissertations and specialist books.

Visit us on the internet:

http://www.grin.com/

http://www.facebook.com/grincom

http://www.twitter.com/grin_com

JIMMA UNIVERSITY

COLLEGE OF AGRICULTURE AND VETERINARY MEDICINE

SCHOOL OF VETERINARY MEDICINE

A REVIEW ON SALMONELLA ENTERITIDIS: TRANSOVARIAL TRANSMISSION MECHANISM IN LAYING CHICKENS

BY

Diriba Taddese Legesse and Minda Asfaw Garesu

August, 29, 2017

JIMMA, ETHIOPIA

TABLE OF CONTENT   PAGES

LIST OF FIGURES

LIST OF ABBREVIATIONS

SPI-1	Salmonella Pathogenicity Island
TTSS	Type III Secretion System
GAP	GTPase-activating protein
NF-T3SS	Necrosis Factors Type III Secretion System
ATPase	Adenosine Triphosphatase
SCV	Salmonella Containing Vacuole
PAMPs	Pathogen Associated Molecular Patterns
DAMPs	Danger-Associated-Molecular Patterns
LPS	Lipopolysaccharides
DNA	Deoxyribonucleic Acid
TLR	Toll-Like Receptor
NF-κB	Nuclear Factor Kappa B
Pro-IL	Proinflammatory Interleukin
IRAK-M	Interleukin Receptor Associated Kinase
NOD	Nucleotide-Binding Oligomerization Domain
NLRs	Nucleotide-Binding OligomerizationDomainlike receptors
FimD	Fimbria D

ACKNOWLEGEMENTS

I would like to extend my gratitude for Jimma University College of Agriculture and Veterinary Medicine for giving me the chance to prepare this review through which I improve my skill of writing scientific prepare.

Finally, I would like to extend my heartfelt thanks to all of my friends for their support in providing me necessary information and constructive comments during preparation of this review.

SUMMARY

Salmonella Enteritidis has been the major cause of food-borne salmonellosis pandemic in humans over e last 20 years, during which contaminated hen's eggs were the most important vehicle of the infection. The main slot of *Salmonella Enteritidis* reserves' is the intestinal tract of chickens and their egg through transovarian transmission route. Hence, the main objective of this manuscript is to review the transovarial transmission mechanism of *Salmonella Enteritidis* in laying chickens. In transovarian transmission, the causative agents could transmit to the offspring following invasion of the reproductive organ. Upon colonizing the reproductive organs, *Salmonella Enteritidis* could invade both phagocytic and non-phagocytic cells in order to bypass the host immune system. In this review, colonization of the ovary, oviduct, vagina, isthmus and magnum by *Salmonella Enteritidis* associated with the respective virulence factors has been discussed in detail. In addition to this, the interaction of the pathogen with the forming egg, its growth within the egg, the role of internal temperature of the egg in multiplication of the bacteria has been conferred critically. Thus, this review paper entitles for the learning of transovarian transmission of *Salmonella Enteritidis* in different reproductive organs of chickens and laid eggs in order to apply a well-coordinated prevention and control methods.

Key words: *Chickens, Eggs, Reproductive Organs, Salmonella Enteritidis, Transovarian Transmission.*

1. INTRODUCTION

The genus *Salmonella* belongs to family Enterobacteriaceae and its classification follows the Kauffmann-White scheme, which groups serotypes according to their somatic, flagella and capsular antigens. The first being subdivided into six subspecies which are designed by Roman numeral, containing more than 2500 antigenically distinct serotype which are a medically important pathogen for both humans and animals (Malony *et al.*, 2011).

The main niche of *Salmonella* servers' is the intestinal tract of humans and farm animals. It can also be present in the intestinal tract of wild birds and their egg, reptiles, and occasionally insects. Feedstuff, soil, bedding, litter, and fecal matter are commonly identified as sources of *Salmonella* contamination in farms (Hoelzer *et al.*, 2011).

Salmonella from fecal contamination can colonizes the gastrointestinal tract of chickens Abulreesh, (2012) and also humans and animals that consume polluted water that shed the bacteria through fecal matter continuing of the cycle of contamination. Yet, there is some consistency in recovery rates of specific serovars (Bailey *et al.*, 2001; Liljebjelke *et al.*, 2005) from these, *S. Enteritidis* became the most frequent serovar reported causing human salmonellosis. From 1985 to 2003 in 75% of *S. Enteritidis* outbreak cases, eggs were confirmed as the primary ingredient or food vehicle of contamination (Liljebjelke *et al.*, 2005). A major outbreak occurred in 1994 where tanker trailers that previously carried *S. Enteritidis* contaminated liquid eggs cause the cross contamination of ice-cream prepared at the same facility (Deligios *et al.*, 2014).

Most commonly, hens are infected with *S. Enteritidis* by vertical transmission through transovarian infection of eggs. *S. Typhimurium* and other serovars usually contaminate eggs externally by penetrating the egg shell (Gantois, 2009). Generally, however it is not yet clear as to which route is most important for *S. Enteritidis* to contaminate the egg contents (Guard-Petter, 2001) there are two possible routes of egg contamination by this agent. These are horizontal transmission (De Reu *et al.*, 2006) and transovarian transmission (Okamura *et al.*, 2001a and b).

The transovarian transmission is the direct contamination of the yolk, albumen, eggshell membranes or eggshells with the *S. Enteritidis* infections originated from the infected reproductive organs before oviposition (Okamura M, *et al.*, 2001a and b). Therefore, the

1

objective of this review is to assess the *Salmonella Enteritidis* transovarial transmission mechanism in layer chickens.

2. MECHANISM OF TRANSOVARIAN TRANSMISSION OF *SALMONELLA ENTERITIDIS* IN LAYING CHICKENS

Transovarian is the transmission of causative agents of disease to offspring following invasion of the reproductive organ. From different causative agents *S. Enteritidis* agent is solitary. In this transmission, this bacterium is introduced from infected reproductive tissues to eggs prior to shell formation. *S. Enteritidis* serotypes associated with poultry reproductive tissues with the intention of public health concern that able to achieve invasion, and as a consequence, may be found more frequently in reproductive tissue (Figure 1) (Mosby, 2009).

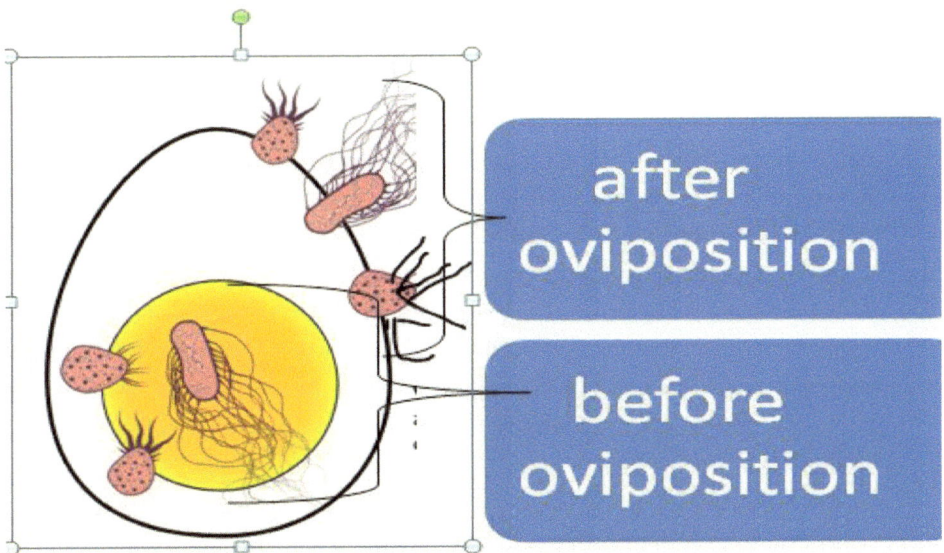

Figure 2: Transovarian and horizontal transmission of *Salmonella Enteritidis*

Source: (Mosby, 2009)

This possible route is by direct contamination of the *S. Enteritidis* infection originating from the reproductive organs like:- ovary, infundibulum, magnum, and isthmus and shell gland with yolk, yolk membranes, albumen, shell membranes and egg shell respectively before oviposition (Figure 2).

The transovarian transmission occurs when *S. Enteritidis* cells migrate to the egg inside of the hen before the egg shell is formed. This is via movement of this cell into the reproductive tract and then enters into the albumen or yolk prior to the egg shell formation (Gantois *et al.*, 2009).

Salmonella Enteritidis is orally taken up by the hen and enters the intestinal tract. Bacteria colonizing the intestinal lumen are able to invade the intestinal epithelial cells (gut colonization). As a consequence, immune cells, more specifically macrophages, are attracted to the site of invasion and enclose the *Salmonella* bacteria. This allows the bacteria to survive and multiply in the intracellular environment of the macrophage. These infected macrophages migrate to the internal organs such as the reproductive organs (systemic spread). *Salmonella* bacteria deposited in the albumen and on the vitelline membrane are able to survive and grow in the antibacterial environment. They are also capable of migrating to and penetrating the vitelline membrane in order to reach the yolk (Gantois *et al.*, 2009).

During the egg formation, the albumen or the egg membranes (rarely the yolk itself) are contaminated as a result of an existing infectious disease of the ovaries or the oviduct. The existing infectious disease of the reproductive organs may originate from systemic infections or it can be an ascending infection from a contaminated cloacae to vagina and then to oviduct. Some bacteria that produce systemic infections *(Salmonella)* are introduced to the hens via the gastrointestinal tract. After oral ingestion, these bacteria colonize several regions of the digestive tract, particularly crop and caeca in the case of *S. Enteritidis* disrupts digestive epithelium, enter the bloodstream and spread through the body of the bird to many organs including the reproductive system Agulles (2014).

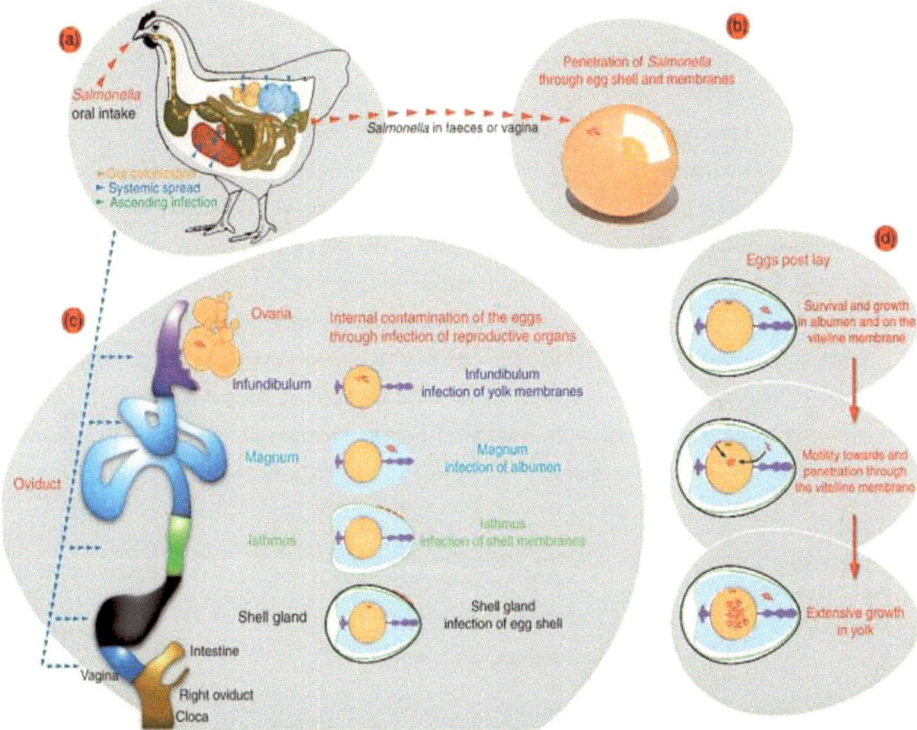

Figure 3: Egg contamination by Pathogenesis of *Salmonella Enteritidis*

Source: Gruenheid and Brett, (2003).

a) Salmonella is orally taken up by the hen and enters the intestinal tract.
b) Egg contamination by Salmonella penetration through the eggshell and shell membranes after outer shell contamination.
c) Direct contamination of the yolk, yolk membranes, albumen, shell membranes and egg shell originating from infection of the ovary, infundibulum, magnum, and isthmus and shell gland, respectively.
d) Salmonella bacteria deposited in the albumen and on the vitelline membrane (Figure 2)

2.1. The Route of Infection and Colonization of the Poultry

Poultry are raised in hen houses that vary in construction, moisture and organic material; they are populated by different pests, such as rodents, insects and wild birds; and poultry are managed with different practices, including the use of molting and biocontainment. Thus, the hen house is not a single environment, but a number of niches in which bacteria survive and multiply. Egg contaminations are prevented in part by stocking the hen house with culture negative chicks from uninfected breeder and multiplier birds (Hoelzer *et al.*, 2011). However, *S. Enteritidis* can be cultured from insect and animal hosts living in and around hen houses, which means that exclusion requires stringent bio containment practices a diversity of environments, living and inanimate, are colonized or infected. Eggs are said to be contaminated rather than infected, as they are not fertile and do not contain living cells. For epidemiological purposes, the route is primarily linear, with humans as the end host. However, transmission of infection from humans to chickens suggests that the route can be cyclical (Figure 3) (Guard-Petter, 2001).

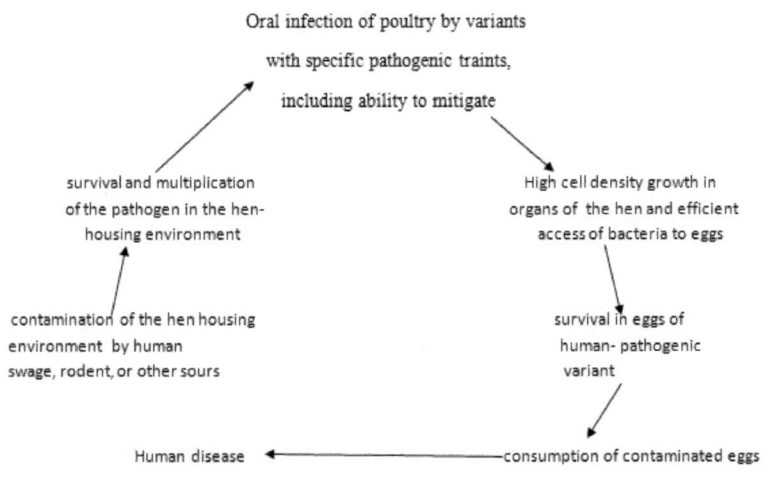

Figure 4: The infection route of *S. Enteritidis*

Source: Guard-Petter, (2001).

2.2. Invasion

Salmonella Enteritidis entry into host cells is mediated by the *Salmonella* pathogenicity island-1 (SPI-1) type III secretion system (TTSS) and its effectors. Membrane attachment to the cortical acting cytoskeleton is loosened by SopB, SopE and SopE2 enhance Cdc42 and Rac1 activity directly by acting as guanine-nucleotide-exchange factors. SipA and SipC alter cytoskeleton structure, SipC by nucleating actin and initiating polymerization and SipA by binding actin and modulating actin bundling. These cytoskeleton rearrangements are down regulated by the GTPase-activating protein (GAP) activity of SptP, which inactivates Cdc42 and Rac. SigD also is involved in sealing invagiating regions of the plasma membrane to form intracellular vacuoles (Figure 4) (Gruenheid *et al*, 2003).

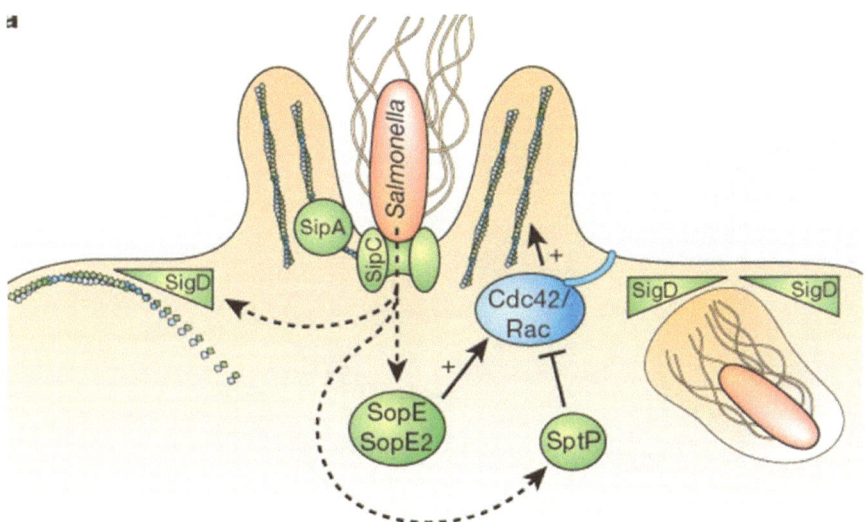

Figure 5: *Salmonella* and its first encounter with the host

Source: Gruenheid *et al.* (2003)

Salmonella pathogenicity island-1(SPI-I) have played a fundamental role in the evolution of the genus *Salmonella*, encodes a type III secretion system including the components of the secretion apparatus effectors proteins, specific chaperones, and virulence gene regulators. The type III systems allow injection of bacterial proteins directly into the cytoplasm of the host cell and they are called "contact-dependent" to reflect this capacity for injection. The structural components of the T3SS apparatus - span both bacterial membranes and the periplasm allow and effectors proteins to be exported in a single step. The secretion apparatus is supplemented by a lanceolate structure protruding from the apparatus and the NF-T3SS has been referred to as a "molecular syringe" (Figure 5) (Galan and Wolf-Watz, 2006).

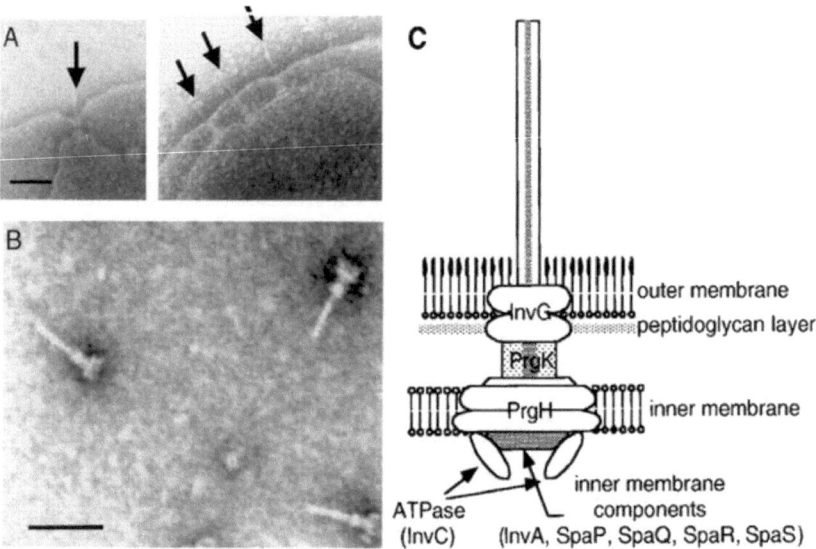

Figure 6: The Type III secretion systems encoded by SPI-I

Source: Galan and Wolf-Watz, (2006)

2.2.1. Invasion of phagocytic and non-phagocytic cells

Salmonella is a facultative intracellular pathogen that can be found in a variety of phagocytic and non-phagocytic cells, in which it is able to survive and replicate. To establish this intracellular niche, the T3SS1 and -2 play a predominant role; key virulence factors are involved in accessing and utilizing these cells. After ingestion, intestinal colonization follows and *Salmonella* enters enterocytes and dendritic cells in the intestinal epithelium (Ibarra and Steele-Mortimer, 2009).

Subsequently, *Salmonella* that reach the submucosa can be internalized by resident macrophages via different mechanisms: by phagocytosis, active invasion using the T3SS1 or T3SS1-independent invasion using fimbriae or other adhesions on the bacterial surface. (1) *Salmonella*-containing-vacuole: - Following internalization *Salmonella* remains within a modified phagosome known as the *Salmonella* containing vacuole (SCV) and injects a limited number of effectors proteins, such as SipA, SipC, SopB/SigD, SodC-1, SopE2, and SptP into the cytoplasm. These effectors cause rearrangements of the actin cytoskeleton and SCV morphology among other changes (Figure.6a) (Gruenheid et al., 2003). (2) Replication within the SCV: - *Salmonella* survives and replicates within the SCV, where it is able to avoid host antimicrobial effectors mechanisms. The T3SS2 is required for systemic virulence in the mouse and survival within macrophages. (3) Transport of *Salmonella* to distant sites: - After penetration of the M cells, the invading microorganisms translocate to the intestinal lymphoid follicles and the draining mesenteric lymph nodes, and some pass on to the reticulo endothelial cells of the liver and spleen. *Salmonella* organisms are able to survive and multiply within the mononuclear phagocytic cells of the lymphoid follicles, liver, and spleen (Figure 6a) (Ibarra and Steele-Mortimer, 2009).

2.2.2. Host pathogen interaction

Simplified scheme of the first encounter between *Salmonella* and the immune system is specified cells such as neutrophils, macrophages, dendritic, phagocytic, and epithelial cells recognize specific pathogen associated molecular patterns (PAMPs) and danger-associated-molecular patterns (DAMPs), there by eliciting an immune response. Pathogen-associated molecular patterns (PAMPs) such as Lipolysaccharides (LPS), flagella, and bacterial Deoxyribonucleic acid (DNA) can trigger Toll-like receptor (TLR) 4, TLR5, and TLR9, respectively.

TLR-induced activation of nuclear factor kappa B (NF-κB) essential for the production of proinflammatory interleukin (pro-IL) 1β, pro-IL-18, is negatively regulated by interleukin receptor associated Kinas (IRAK-M) (Fig.5.b) (Crawford *et al.*, 2010).

The nucleotide-binding oligomerization domain -like receptors (NLRs) is situated in the cytosol and can also recognize PAMPs. However, NLRP3 is triggered by a different, yet unknown, mechanism, although DAMPs are thought to play a crucial role. TLR; LPS; NF-κB, regulated nuclear factor kappa-light-chain-enhancer of activated B cells; IRAK-M, IL-1R-assiociated kinase-M; IL, Interleukin; ASC, apoptotic spick protein containing a caspase recruitment domain; NLR, nucleotide-binding oligomerization domain(NOD) like receptors (including NLRP3 and NLRC4); MyD88, myeloid differentiation primary response gene (Figure.6b) (Crawford *et al.*, 2010).

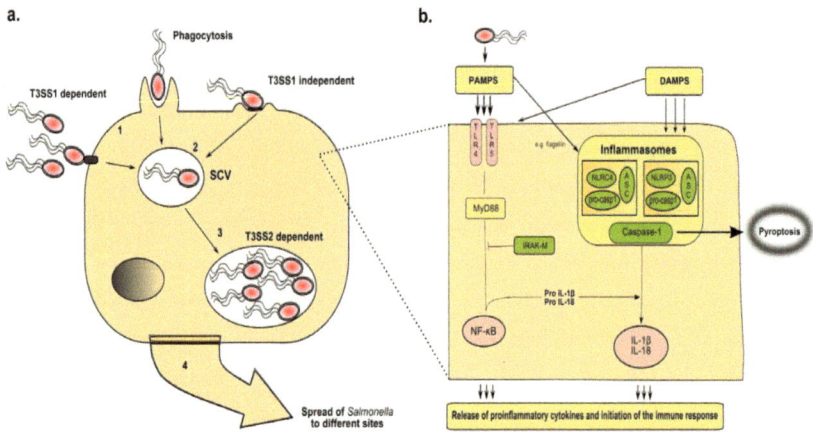

Figure 7: *Salmonella* invasion to phagocytic and non-phagocytic cells and host–pathogen interaction

Source: Crawford *et al.* (2010).

2.2.3. Infection of epithelial cells of the lower intestine and macrophages by *Salmonella Enteritidis*

(A) The complex membrane structure of *Salmonella* allows it to survive until reaching the epithelial cell wall of the host in the lower intestine.

(B) *Salmonella* then translocate across M cells of Peyer's patches or actively invade epithelial cells by the secretion of effectors proteins through the SPI-1 encoded T3SS-1.

(C) (i) After crossing the epithelial barrier, *Salmonella* are engulfed by proximal macrophages that will secrete effectors proteins into the cytosol of the cell via the SPI-2 encoded T3SS- 2 and prevent fusion of the phagosome with the lysosome.

(ii) Within the SCV, *Salmonella* will proliferate resulting in cytokine secretion by the macrophage.

(iii) Finally, the macrophage will undergo apoptosis, and *Salmonella* will escape the cell to basolaterally reinvade epithelial cells or other phagocytic cells of the host innate immune system (Figure 7) (Hurley *et al.,* 2014).

A

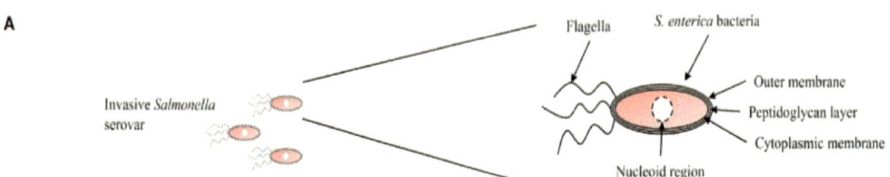

Invasive *Salmonella* serovar

Flagella   *S. enterica* bacteria

Outer membrane

Peptidoglycan layer

Cytoplasmic membrane

Nucleoid region

B

Effector secretion through SPI-1 associated T3SS

SipA, SipB SopB, SopD, SopE, SopE2

Translocation across epithelial barrier

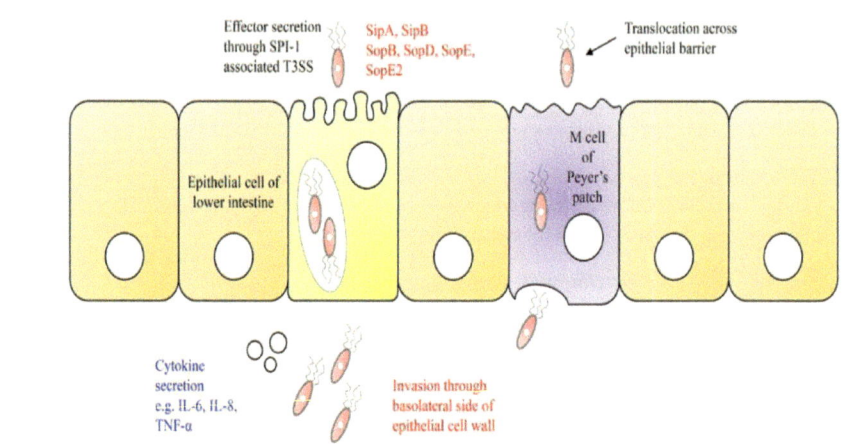

Epithelial cell of lower intestine

M cell of Peyer's patch

Cytokine secretion e.g. IL-6, IL-8, TNF-α

Invasion through basolateral side of epithelial cell wall

C

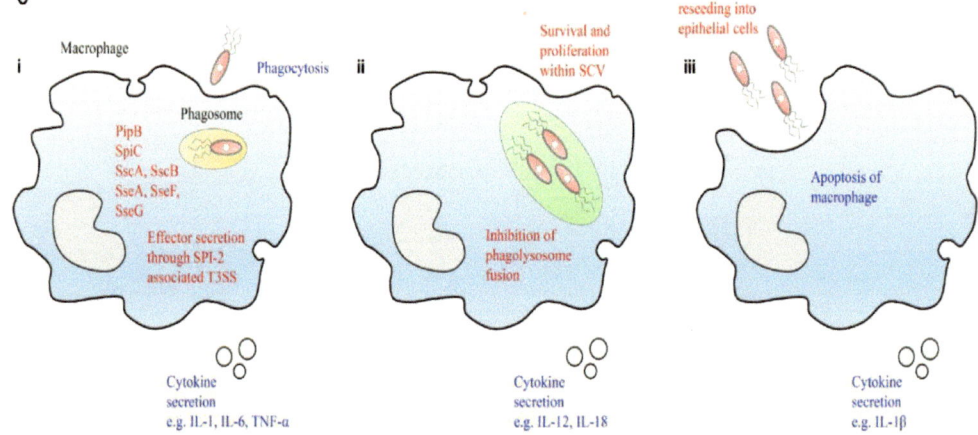

Basolateral reseeding into epithelial cells

Macrophage

i

Phagocytosis

ii

Survival and proliferation within SCV

iii

Phagosome

PipB
SpiC
SscA, SscB
SseA, SseF,
SseG

Effector secretion through SPI-2 associated T3SS

Inhibition of phagolysosome fusion

Apoptosis of macrophage

Cytokine secretion e.g. IL-1, IL-6, TNF-α

Cytokine secretion e.g. IL-12, IL-18

Cytokine secretion e.g. IL-1β

12

Figure 8: Schematic illustration of the infection of epithelial cells of the lower intestine and macrophages by *Salmonella Enteritides*

Source: Hurley *et al.* (2014)

2.3. Colonization of the Reproductive Organs

Several lines of evidence support the view that egg contamination with *S. Enteritides* is more likely to take place during the formation of the egg in the reproductive organs than by eggshell penetration. In several studies, *S. Enteritides* was isolated from the reproductive tissue of infected birds, in the absence of intestinal colonization. Moreover, *S. Enteritides* is capable of persistence in reproductive tissues of naturally and experimentally infected hens, even though the animals generate an innate and adaptive immune response to the infection, indicating that the bacteria can reside intracellular and escape the host defense mechanisms. The deposition of *Salmonella* inside eggs is thus most likely a consequence of reproductive tissue colonization in infected laying hens (Gast & Holt, 2000).

Very little is known, however, about the exact site in reproductive tissues where the bacteria reside and the bacterial and host factors that play a role in the association between the reproductive tissue and *Salmonella*. The oviduct can be subdivided into five functional regions. Starting from the ovary, there are the infundibulum, magnum, isthmus, uterus and vagina. The infundibulum captures the ovulatory follicles, the magnum produces the albumen, the isthmus deposits the eggshell membranes, the uterus forms the eggshell and the vagina is involved in oviposition (Bohez *et al.*, 2008).

According to most authors, the albumen is most frequently contaminated, pointing to the oviduct tissue as the colonization site. However, some studies found the yolk to be primarily contaminated, suggesting the ovary to be the primary colonization site (Bohez *et al.*, 2008). It is thus difficult, based on the contamination site in eggs, to predict the most important colonization site of *Salmonella* in the reproductive tract. However, it would be reasonable to suggest that, given that *S. Enteritides* can be isolated from all sites in the hen reproductive tract, that contamination of any part of the egg is possible (Gast and Holt, 2000; Bohez *et al.*, 2008).

It is generally believed that colonization of the reproductive organs is a consequence of systemic spread of *Salmonella* from the intestine. Invasion in the intestinal epithelial cells triggers

13

infiltration of immune cells, mainly macrophages, resulting in the uptake of bacteria by these cells.

Because of its capability to survive and replicate in the immune cells, bacteria carried in the macrophages are spread within the host, resulting in colonization of the reproductive organs (Howard *et al.*, 2005).

Salmonella pathogenicity island-2 (SPI-2) is essential in the ability to spread within the host and to cause a systemic infection. Using a deletion mutant in the regulator of SPI-2,it was shown that after intravenous infection of laying hens, the bacterial numbers of the mutant were significantly lower in the oviducts and the ovaries as compared with the wild-type strain. These reduced colony counts in the reproductive organs point to a role for SPI-2 in the spread or the colonization of the reproductive tract tissues (Gast and Holt, 2000).

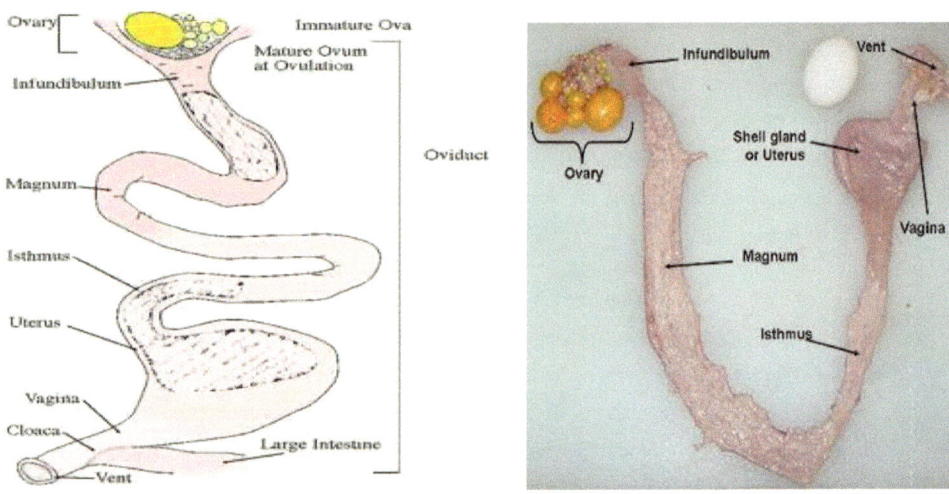

Figure 9 : Reproductive Organs of Hen

Source: Gast and Holt, (2000)

2.3.1. Colonization of the ovary

The extensive permeability of the vascular endothelia observed in the ovary may contribute to the high colonization rate at this site. In the majority of experimental studies in laying hens, a higher frequency of ovary colonization is reported, compared with the frequency of recovery from the oviduct. Therefore, it is strongly believed that *S. Enteritides* must interact with the cellular components of the pre-ovulatory follicles (Howard *et al.*, 2005). It was indeed shown that *S. Enteritides* can attach to developing and mature follicular granulosa cells exhibiting different attachment patterns. Higher bacterial numbers in the membranes of the preovulatory follicles than in the yolk itself suggest that during transovarian transmission, *S. Enteritides* remains attached to the egg vitelline membranes (Figure 2) (Gast *et al.*, 2007).

A previous study has also suggested that yolk contamination is more often associated with the vitelline membrane than with the interior yolk contents. It has been noticed that in vitro attachment of *S. Enteritides* to granulosa cells may involve binding to fibronectin. Furthermore, a major role of the type 1 fimbriae in the attachment process was suggested because the in vitro attachment of *S. Enteritides* to granulosa cells was inhibited by pre incubation of the cells with purified fimbrial preparation. There are also indications that *Salmonella* can invade and multiply in granulosa cells (Gast and Holt, 2000) compared the ability of *Salmonella* to invade ovarian follicles at different stages of follicular maturity in vitro: the small white follicles (immature) were more susceptible to *Salmonella* invasion than the more mature small and large yellow ones.

These authors believe that the penetration of immature follicles has practical implications because it can lead to contamination of eggs after maturation and can cause continuous transovarian infection of eggs throughout the reproductive cycle. This statement is, however, questionable because not all small white follicles will mature and because the extensive growth of *Salmonella* in the nutrient-rich follicles will most likely lead to their degeneration. Studies comparing invasion of the serotypes *Enteritidis* and *Typhimurium* in ovarian follicles in vitro yielded conflicting results. Based on the fact that systemic fspread is a characteristic of most *Salmonella* serotypes, it is believed that ovarian colonization is not a specific trait allowing the serotype *Enteritidis* to contaminate eggs (Howard *et al.*, 2005).

15

However, the possibility that *S. Enteritides* has a specific ability to interact and invade the preovulatory follicles cannot be ruled out. A large-scale study using multiple strains from different *Salmonella* serotypes should be carried out in order to provide more information regarding the serotype specificity of ovarian colonization and persistence (Mizumoto *et al.*, 2005). High levels of nutrients are available to bacteria invading ovarian follicles. Therefore, it is to be expected that this should lead to extensive replication of the bacteria, almost inevitably resulting in follicular degeneration. Because this is not a common phenomenon in naturally infected laying hens, as the laying percentage is usually not reduced, follicle colonization is not believed to be an important source of egg contamination, although this is under debate (Howard *et al.*, 2005).

2.3.2. Colonization of the oviduct

Although several studies reported the vitelline membrane as the most common site of *Salmonella* contamination other reports point to albumen as the principal site of contamination in eggs indicating that *S. Enteritides* is colonizing oviduct tissues observed that developing eggs in a highly contaminated oviduct are likely to be *Salmonella* positive. Colonization of the reproductive tract can be the result of an ascending infection from the cloaca (a descending infection from the ovary and/or a systemic spread of *Salmonella*. Depending on the site of contamination, i.e. the vagina, isthmus and magnum, *Salmonella* could be incorporated into the eggshell, the eggshell membranes or the albumen (Figure 2) (Gast and Holt, 2000a).

2.3.3. Vaginal colonization

Several authors have focused on the role of the vagina in the production of *S. Enteritides* - contaminated eggs. It is believed that intravaginal infection tends to ascend only to the lower parts of the oviduct because *Salmonella* is rarely recovered from the ovary and the upper oviduct in intravaginally inoculated hens (Okamura, *et al.*, 2001b). Several studies obtained high egg contamination rates after intravaginal infection, indicating a high risk of contamination (primarily eggshell contamination) as the egg passes through a heavily colonized vagina. When the egg is laid, penetration through the eggshell can occur, due to suction of the organisms into eggs under the negative pressure caused by cooling of the egg (Mizumoto *et al.*, 2005).

In spite of the fact that it is difficult to distinguish between contamination during formation of the egg or after oviposition, internal egg contamination after vaginal colonization most likely occurs after penetration of the eggshell and not by internal contamination following ascending infection of the upper oviduct, although this cannot be ruled out. In a comparative study with six different *Salmonella* serotypes, significantly higher numbers of *S. Enteritides* were recovered from the vagina in comparison with strains belonging to other serotypes after intravaginal inoculation (Buck *et al.*, 2004).

The same authors suggested that a higher ability of the serotype *Enteritidis* to attach to the vaginal epithelium. It was also noticed so as to the rank order of the *Salmonella* invasiveness in vaginal epithelium was dependent on the lippolysaccharide type, namely lippolysaccharide type O9 (*S. Enteritides*)>lippolysaccharide type O4 (*Salmonella Typhimurium, Salmonella Heidelberg* and *Salmonella Agona*)>lippolysaccharide type O7 (*Salmonella Montevideo* and *Salmonella Infants*) and lippolysaccharide type O8 (Mizumoto *et al.*, 2005).

2.3.4. Isthmus and magnum colonization

It is clear that different segments of the oviduct can be colonized by *S. Enteritidis* using different infection models, the tubular glands of the isthmus were identified as the predominant colonization site of *S. Enteritides* in the oviduct by colonization of the isthmus can result in contaminated eggshell membranes. These observations are in accordance with other experimental studies (Okamura *et al.*, 2001).

In principle, eggshell membrane contamination can also be a consequence of penetration of *Salmonella* bacteria after deposition on the shell during the passage through the vagina rather than direct contamination of the eggshell membranes during passage through the isthmus. In addition, when culturing the eggshell and egg contents separately, some albumen sticks to the eggshell, making the interpretations of the shell membranes as the site of egg contamination even more complex (Mizumoto *et al.*, 2005).

Numerous studies suggest that *S. Enteritides* most frequently migrates into eggs through the upper oviduct. Detection of   S. *Enteritides* associated with discharging cells of the upper and lower magnum by immune histochemical staining is in agreement with the hypothesis that the pathogen may contaminate forming eggs through the albumen (Buck *et al.*, 2004).

Recently, the abilities to invade and proliferate in isthmus and magnum oviduct cells of different *Salmonella* serotypes were assessed using a tubular gland cell primary culture model. All serotypes tested were equally able to invade and proliferate in the glandular epithelial cells, suggesting that invasion and proliferation in oviduct cells is most likely not a unique characteristic of the serotype *Enteritidis* (Gantois *et al.*, 2008).

Also *Salmonella* serotype *Enteritidis* and *Typhimurium* strain colonized the oviduct to higher levels than strains belonging to the serotypes Heidelberg, Virchow and Hadar, even if all serotypes invaded oviduct cells *in vitro*. Demonstrating that of six serotypes, only *Enteritidis* and *Typhimurium* were able to colonize the reproductive organs at days 4 and 7 post inoculation. One-day-old chicks that were orally infected with the chicken-adapted *Salmonella* Pullorum produced a high amount of contaminated eggs (6.5%) during the period of sexual maturity as a consequence of reproductive organ colonization. Isolates of *S* Enteritides and *Salmonella* Pullorum, together with isolates of *Salmonella Gallinarum* and *Salmonella Dublin*, form a related strain cluster that share the same lippolysaccharide-based O-antigen structure (O-1, 9, 12, characteristic of sero group D) (Buck *et al.*, 2004).

Comparative genome analysis of *S. Enteritidis* and *Salmonella Gallinarum* indicated that these serotypes are highly related and that *Salmonella Gallinarum* may be a direct descendant of *S. Enteritidis*. It can be speculated that these two serotypes harbour the same characteristics, allowing them to efficiently contaminate eggs, but this is not clear (Gantois *et al.*, 2008).

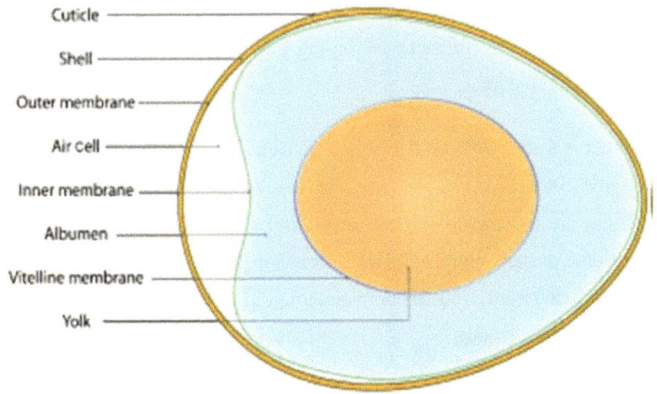

Cuticle
Shell
Outer membrane
Air cell
Inner membrane
Albumen
Vitelline membrane
Yolk

Figure 10: Schematic representation of the egg structure

Source: Buck *et al.* (2004).

2.4. Virulence Factors Associated with Oviduct Colonization

Contaminated laying hens with a fimbria D (fimD) mutant of *S. Enteritidis* resulted in heavier and more frequently contaminated internal organs. This may be due to the effect of the afimbriate state on bacteraemia. Bacteraemia in the laying hens after infection with the *fimD* mutant bacteria was more extensive and longer lasting than after infection with the wild type. The oviduct was more frequently infected by the mutant strain (Parker *et al.*, 2002). Possibly, the higher incidence of the mutant bacteria in the blood may give rise to some incidental isolation of *Salmonella* from the oviduct. However, the higher frequency of infection of the oviduct tissue samples by the mutant strain corresponded with the higher number of isolations of the mutant strain from the oviduct lumen swabs, indicating that the bacteria were actually colonizing the oviduct (Buck *et al.*, 2004).

In order to gain a better understanding of the molecular mechanisms allowing the serotype *Enteritidis* to interact with the hen's reproductive tract and to adapt to this particular ecological niche, a genome-wide screen was carried out by (Gantois *et al.* 2008) to identify genes expressed in the oviduct, using *in vivo* expression technology.

19

This can identified the genes involved in cell wall integrity, regulation of fimbrial operons, amino acid and nucleic acid metabolism, stress response and motility as being highly induced during colonization of the reproductive tract.

This indicates that the oviduct is a stressful and damaging environment for *Salmonella* bacteria, but it also indicates that the bacteria can counteract this by stress-induced protective and reparative responses, enabling the bacteria to survive in the hostile environment and/or escape the host defense reactions. In the present study, *S. Enteritidis* lacking type 1 fimbriae were found to be less capable of contaminating eggs, and the contamination of shell and shell membranes was significantly reduced (Buck *et al.,*2004).

There is mounting evidence that lipolysaccharide is also of particular importance for *S. Enteritidis* persistence in the reproductive tracts tissues. Lipolysaccharide is a major component of the outer membrane of Gram-negative bacteria and a prime target for recognition by the innate immune system. At least two different functions have been attributed to lipolysaccharides with respect to persistent reproductive tract infection. It has been suggested that the composition of lipolysaccharides is important in determining the survival of *S. Enteritides* in avian macrophages and these cells may be a site where *S. Enteritides* resides in the oviduct (He *et al.*, 2006).

Different levels of attachment of different *Salmonella* serotypes to chicken vaginal explants possibly also involve a role of the lipolysaccharide structure. Furthermore, it has been shown that high-molecular-weight lipolysaccharide in *S. Enteritides* is correlated with increased egg contamination although the exact role of high-molecular-weight lipolysaccharide is not yet known, its presence has been correlated with an unusual pathology of the reproductive tract, even though this was not reflected in higher egg contamination (Parker *et al.*, 2002).

The type 3 secretion systems-1 and -2 (T3SS-1 and T3SS-2) may also play a role in egg contamination. T3SS-1 is mainly associated with bacterial invasion of the intestinal epithelium via the concerted action of effectors proteins while T3SS-2 is responsible for the establishment of systemic infection by promoting the intracellular survival of *Salmonella* in macrophages, as mentioned earlier. The first to confirm the pathogenic role of T3SS-1 and T3SS-2 effectors in *S. Enteritidis* is for invasion and intracellular survival in the epithelial cell of chicken oviducts. It is

20

believed that invasion and survival in tubular gland cells of the oviduct is not specific for serotype *Enteritidis* (Gantois *et al.*, 2008).

Most likely, functions exerted by T3SS-1 and T3SS-2 are also required by *Salmonella* serotypes other than *Enteritidis* to invade and survive inside chicken oviduct epithelial cells. Furthermore, a recent study suggested that inactivation of *ssrA*, a regulator of T3SS-2, rendered *S. Enteritidis* unable to colonize the chicken reproductive tract successfully (Bohez *et al.*, 2008).

Meanwhile, it has become clear that the process of oviduct colonization is complex and depends on many factors including fimbriae, flagellae, lippolysaccharide, cell wall structure, and stress tolerance. Although most, if not all, bacterial factors, shown to play a role in reproductive tract colonization, are not specific to the serotype *Enteritidis*, a unique regulation of these known virulence factors in the reproductive tract environment could be one plausible explanation for the epidemiological association with hen's eggs. This, however, has not been shown yet (Bohez *et al.*, 2008).

It was demonstrated that repeated *in vivo* passages through the reproductive tissues of chickens increase the ability of an *S. Enteritides* strain to induce internal egg contamination, whereas serial passage through the liver and the spleen did not affect the ability of the strain to cause egg contamination. This is an indication that interaction of *S. Enteritidis* with the reproductive tissues may either induce or select for the expression of microbial properties important for egg contamination. The complementarily between phenotypic traits with relevance for colonization and survival in different tissues may allow *S. Enteritidis* to traverse the complex series of events between the introduction of infection and the deposition inside eggs (Gantois *et al.*, 2009).

2.5. The Interaction between *Salmonella Enteritidis* and the Forming Egg

Egg contamination associated with *S. Enteritidis* is believed to occur before deposition of the shell by internal (vertical) transmission to the contents of the egg (yolk or albumen) via the reproductive tract (Figure 2). It cannot be ruled out that *S. Enteritidis* actively promotes access to the egg by penetration of a marginally faulty shell that excludes most other bacteria. Once inside the egg, bacteria face an inhospitable environment. Egg white is rich in lysozyme and lacks available iron has antibodies. These factors help to limit the growth of bacteria in eggs, although

21

on occasion eggs with very high numbers of bacteria are detected. It is conceivable that some variants of *S. enteritidis* are more adapted for growth and survival in eggs (Guard-Petter, 2001).

2.6. Growth of *Salmonella Enteritidis* in Eggs

Salmonella Enteritidis is believed to grow at differing rates depending on where in the egg initial contamination occurs. A series of contamination events, *S. Enteritidis*, were envisioned at different sites of the egg, or egg compartments, as shell eggs develop within the hen. These contamination events are summarized as follows: Eaf, contamination of albumen far from the yolk; Eac, contamination of albumen close to the yolk; Ev, contamination of the vitelline membrane of the yolk; and Ey, contamination of the yolk. So modeling *S. Enteritidis* growth in albumen depending on site and distance from the yolk (Eac and Eaf), and on the vitelline membrane of the yolk (Humphrey and Whitehead, 2009).

2.7. Internal Temperature of the Egg

The internal temperature of eggs at laying was approximately 99 °F (37 °C), which is the physiological temperature of the hen. Subsequent cooling or warming of the eggs is controlled by the ambient air temperature, storage time, and the cooling rate. The packaging (carton, boxed, stacked in the interior of a pallet) and other factors such as air circulation within the storage area can also influence the egg temperature. The internal temperature is estimated for any storage time by a simplified un-steady-state heat transfer relationship (Whiting and Buchanan, 2007).

3. CONCLUSION AND RECOMMENDATIONS

Generally Salmonella serovars are resilient microorganisms with a complex genomic system that makes the organism able to react to different harsh environmental conditions at the farm, during processing and in the gastrointestinal tract. Evidence is accumulating that contamination of the eggs is not only by penetration through the shell, but also by passage from the hen's intestinal tract to the reproductive tract and from there incorporation into the forming egg on the vitelline membrane, in the egg. The bacteria directly contaminate the yolk, yolk membranes, albumen, shell membranes and egg shell originating from infection of the ovary, infundibulum, magnum, isthmus and shell gland, respectively. They are also capable of migrating to and penetrating the vitelline membrane in order to reach the yolk. Following to reaching this rich environment, they can grow widely and recycle the transition. This situation is associated with agent virulence factors and more frequently infected of oviduct by the mutant strain.

Based on the above concluding remarks, the following recommendations are forwarded:

- For a better understanding of the molecular mechanisms allowing the serotype *Enteritidis* to interact with the hen's reproductive tract, pioneering study has to be conducted by collecting sample from different reproductive organs in order to grasp the route of transmission
- Good manufacturing and handling practices should be under taken by eggs producer to minimize the potential risk of *Salmonella Enteritidis* infection due to the consumption of egg and egg products
- Business operators, producer, consumers and food handlers should be advised for the establishment of good hygiene housing and outline the safe procedure to control the transitions of this agent
- In order to design and utilize effective *Salmonella Enteritidis* vaccines in Ethiopia, further in-depth investigation on isolation and molecular characterization has to be conducted

4. REFERENCES

Abulreesh, H. H. (2012) Salmonellae in the environment, in Salmonella distribution, adaptation, control measures and molecular technologies, Eds., Pp. 19-50.

Agulles, T. M. (2014): How egg quality impacts the health of day-one-chicks? *Poult.Fish Wildl. Sci.*,**2**: 124. doi: 1-3.

Bailey, J. S., Stern, N. J. & Fedorka-Cray, P. (2001): Sources and movement of Salmonella through integrated poultry operations: a multistate epidemiological investigation. *Food Protection,* **64** (11): 1690-1697.

Bohez, L., Gantois, I., Ducatelle, R., Pasmans, F., Dewulf,J,. Haesebrouck, F. & Van Immerseel ,F. (2008): The *salmonella* pathogenicity island 2 regulator SsrA promotes reproductive tract   but not intestinal colonization in chickens. *Vet.Microbiol.*,**126**:216-224.

Crawford, R W., Rosales-Reyes, R., Ramirez-Aguilar MdeL, Chapa-Azuela, O. & Alpuche-Aranda, C. (2010): Gallstones play a significant role in *salmonella* spp. gallbladder colonization   and carriage. *Proc Natl. Acad. Sci.,* **107**: 4353-4358.

Buck, De J., Pasmans, F., Van Immerseel, F., Haesebrouck, F., &Ducatelle, R. (2004): Tubular glands of the isthmus is the predominant colonization site of *salmonella enteritidis* in the upper oviduct of laying hens. *Poultry Sci,* **83**: 352-358.

De Reu, K., Grijspeerdt, K., Messens,W., Heyndrickw, M., Uyttendaele, M., Debevere, J., & Herman, L. (2006): Eggshell factors influencing eggshell penetration and whole egg contamination by different bacteria, including *Salmonella Enteritidis. Int. J. food Microbiol.*,**112** (3): 253-260.

Deligios, M., Bacciu, D. & Deriu, E. (2014): Draft genome sequence of the host-restricted Salmonella entericaserovarabortusovis strain SS44.*Genome Announcements,* **2**(2) v Article ID e00261-214.

Galan, JE. &, Wolf-Watz, H. (2006): Protein delivery into eukaryotic cells by type III secretion machines. *Nature* **444** (7119): 567-573.

Gantois, I., Ducatelle, R., Pasmans, F., &Haesebrouck, F. & Gast, R. (2009): Mechanisms of egg contamination by *Salmonella Enteritidis. FEMS Microbiol. Rev.,* **33**: 718-738.

Gantois, I., Eeckhaut,V., Pasmans, F., Haesebrouck, F., Ducatelle, R., & Van Immerseel, F. (2008): A comparative study on the pathogenesis of egg contamination by different serotypes of *Salmonella. Avian Pathol,* **37**:399-406.

Gast, RK & Holt, PS. (2000): Deposition of phage type 4 and 13a *Salmonella Enteritidis* strains in the yolk and albumen of eggs lay by experimentally infected hens. *Avian Dis.,* **44**: 706-710.

Gast, R. K., Guraya, R., Guard-Bouldin, J., Holt,PS., & Moore, RW. (2007) Colonization of specific regions of the reproductive tract and deposition at different locations inside eggs laid by hens infected with *Salmonella Enteritidis* or *Salmonella Heidelberg. Avian Dis.,* **51**: 40-44.

Gruenheid, S. Brett & Finlay, B. B. (2003) Microbial pathogenesis and cytoskeletal function. *Nature,* **422**:775-781.

Guard-Petter, J. (2001) The chicken, the egg and *Salmonella Enteritidis. Environ Micr,* 421-430.

Guard-Petter, J. (2001) The review highlights the stages of transmission and discusses evidence that altered bacterial growth patterns and specific cell surface. V: **3** Pp. 421-430

He, H., Genovese, K.J., Nisbet, D. J. & Kogut, M.H. (2006) Involvement of phosphatidylinositol- phospholipase C in immune response to *Salmonella* lipopolysaccharide in chicken macrophage cells (HD11). *Int. Immuno. Pharmaco.,* **16**:1780-1787.

Hoelzer, K., Switt, A. I. M. & Wiedmann, M. (2011) Animal contact as a source of human non-typhoidal salmonellosis. *Vet. Res.,* **42**(1), article 34.

Howard, Z. R., Moore, R. W., Zabala-Diaz, I. B., Landers, K. L., Byrd, J. A., Kubena, L. F., Nisbet, D. J., Birkhold, S. G., & Ricke, S. C. (2005) Ovarian laying hen follicular maturation and in vitro *Salmonella* internalization. *Vet Microbiol.,* **108**: 95-100.

Humphrey, T. J & Whitehead, A. (2009) Egg age and the growth of *Salmonella enteritidis* PT4 in egg contents. *Epidemiol. Infect.,* **111**:209-219.

Hurley, D., Mc Cusker, M. P., Fanning, S., & Martins, M. (2014) Salmonella–host interactions modulation of the host innate immune system., *Frontiers Immunol,***5**: 481-489.

Ibarra, J. A. & Steele-Mortimer, O. (2009): *Salmonella* the ultimate insider *Salmonella* virulence factors that modulate intracellular survival. *Cell Microbiol.,* **11**: 1579-1586.

Liljebjelke, K. A. & Hofacre, C. L. (2005) Vertical and horizontal transmission of *Salmonella* within integrated broiler production system, *Foodborne Pathogens Dis.,* **2**: 90-102.

Malony, B., Hauser, E. & Dieckmann, R. (2011) New approaches in subspecies-level *Salmonella* classification in S*almonella* from genome to function, S. Porwollik, Ed., Pp.1-23, *Academic Press, Norfolk, UK.*

Mizumoto, N., Sasai K., Tani, H. & Baba, E. (2005) Specific adhesion and invasion of *Salmonella Enteritidis* in the vagina of laying hens. *Vet .Microbiol,* 111: 99-105.

Mosby's (2009): Medical dictionary: transovarial transmission.Medical dictionary, 8th Edition, Retrieved June 4, 2017.

Okamura, M., Kamijima, Y., Miyamoto, T., Tani, H., Sasai, K. & Baba, E. (2001) Differences among six *Salmonella* serovars in abilities to colonize reproductive organs and to contaminate   eggs in laying hens. *Avian Dis,* 45: 61-69.

Okamura, M., Miyamoto, T., Kamijima, Y., Tani, H., Sasai, K. & Baba, E. (2001) Differences in abilities to colonize reproductive organs and to contaminate eggs in intravaginally inoculated hens and in vitro adherences to vaginal explants between *Salmonella Enteritidis* and other *Salmonella*s erovars. *Avian Dis,* 45: 962-971.

Parker, C. T., Harmon, B. & Guard-Petter, J. (2002) Mitigation of avian reproductive tract functions by *Salmonella Enteritidis* producing high-molecular-mass lipopolysaccharide *Environ. Microbio.,* 14: 538-545.

Whiting, R. C. & Buchanan, R. L. (2007) Progress in microbiological modeling and risk assessment In Food Microbiology*:* Fundamentals and Frontiers, *Third Edition American Society of Microbiology*, Pp. 953-969.

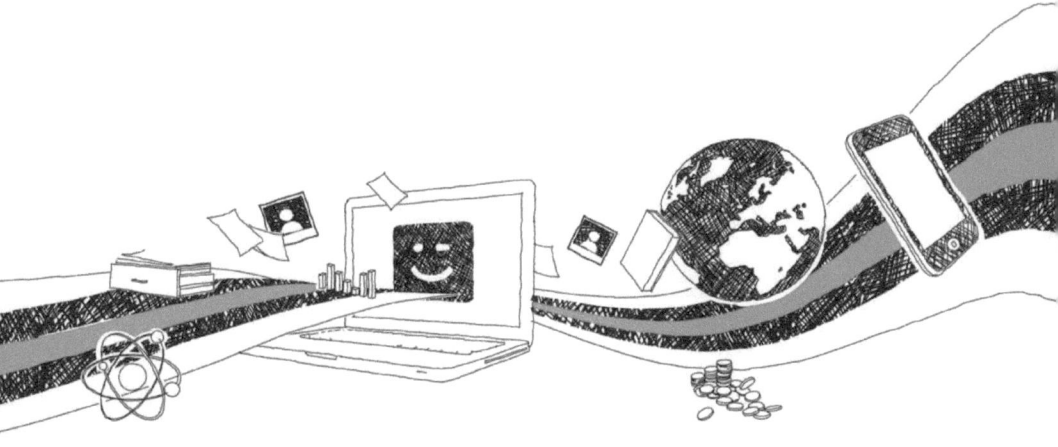
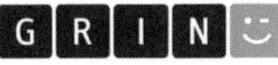